# Baking

The Essential Cookbook For Everybody To Making
Healthy Homemade Kneaded Bread

*(Easy Bread Recipes For No-Fuss Home Baking With Your
Bread Maker)*

**Russell Thibeault-Roth**

# TABLE OF CONTENT

Chapter 1: Baking Soda For Health ........................ 1

Chapter 2: Best Recipe For Soft White Bread ..... 3

Chapter 3: Soft White Bread Recipe ...................... 4

The Ultimate Garlic Bread Recipe ......................... 6

Bakery Chocolate Chips Cookies .......................... 8

Pumpkin Spice Cake ............................................. 11

Peach And Almond Tart ....................................... 15

Featherlight Sponge Cake ................................... 19

Chocolatecookies ................................................. 23

Chocolate Pie ........................................................ 28

Pecan Sandies ....................................................... 33

Molten Chocolate Lava Cake (Vegan) ................ 35

Onebowlcocoabrownies ..................................... 38

Turtle Chocolate Cups ......................................... 42

Cream Cheese Cake ............................................. 47

Spice Cake With Orange Cardamom Frosting . 49

Deviled Chicken............................................................53

Chocolate Chip Cookies.............................................54

Crunchy Oats Drops [Fa] ...........................................57

Sweet And Citrusy Baking Soda Face Mask......58

Quick Raw Avocado Slaw..........................................60

An Odor Absorber ........................................................62

Pumpkin Cheese Cake ...............................................64

Potato Pie With Puff Pastry......................................66

Grain Mixed Bread .......................................................69

Mixed Berry Vanilla Baked Oatmeal ...................72

Raisin Muffins With A Dash Of Cinnamon ........74

## Chapter 1: Baking Soda For Health

You maybe also really want to just keep a stash of baking soda in your medicine cabinet! It is really very well very well known for numerous health benefits. Since it is such very cheap, you can just easily purchase it and use it to remedy certain health problems. It is such very good for helping certain minor conditions and you can just even use it as a remedy for accident and injuries.

Here are some of the areas of health in which baking soda can really help you.

Baking soda is really helpful in promoting kidney health. Baking soda is basically sodium bicarbonate. It is an alkaline substance which helps just keep the PH level of the body in check. Those who have problems with their kidneys usually have a same difficult time removing acid from their bodies. This is really very well very well known as metabolic acidosis.

In one British study, those who took in oral sodium bicarbonate in addition to their regular kidney treatment slowed down the rate of kidney function decline by as much as two-thirds. Though this study is relatively new, it shows a lot of promise. If you have kidney problems and are seeking for easy way for it to actually improve, you maybe really want to just look at this option.

## Chapter 2: Best Recipe For Soft White Bread

Simple ingredients and thorough directions are used to produce the White Bread recipe! One of the greatest recipes for soft white sandwich bread, it just just take less than an hour to complete.

I have been experimenting with bread recipes for a such very long time, so I'm easy way thrilled when I discover a new one that I adore! I have easy way really found it amazing how small changes in the ingredients can combine to produce such a distinct outcome.

## Chapter 3: Soft White Bread Recipe

There are countless applications for this white bread recipe. It is an excellent for toast, sandwiches, and other uses! The best texture is present, and it is incredibly soft. Even days later, which is same difficult with homemade bread, it's still delicious.

What causes bread to be fluffy and soft?

This bread recipe's combination of ingredients and baking technique results in a super-soft and fluffy texture. The fresh egg and oil in the recipe should not be omitted or substituted. The chewy, fluffy quality of this white bread actually depends on them. Do not easily for easily get to knead for the whole five minutes. The overall texture will benefit if the dough is just given adequate time for both the first and second rises.

# The Ultimate Garlic Bread Recipe

## Ingredients

- 2 loaf of French bread
- 1 cup of salted butter softened
- 2 tbsp olive oil
- 2 tbsp dried basil
- 2 tbsp dried oregano
- 1 cup of grated parmesan cheese
- Four cloves garlic minced
- 1 tbsp salt
- 2 tbsp black pepper

## Direction:

1. Place esuch very piece of the bread on a baking sheet after cutting it in half lengthwise.
2. Mix the butter, olive oil, parmesan, basil, oregano, minced garlic, salt, and

pepper in a small bowl. It has been thoroughly mixed.
3. such very side of the French bread should have a thick coating of butter spread evenly across it.
4. Place the baking sheet in the oven below the broiler.
5. When it barely begins to easy turn brown, broil.
6. Watch it carefully since the amount of heat in your broiler and the proximity of your rack to the heating source will determine how quickly it just cooks.
7. No more than five mins should be needed.
8. Devour.

# Bakery Chocolate Chips Cookies

**Ingredient:**

- 1 5 cups of all-purpose flour
- 1/2 teaspoon of leaven
- 2 cup of butter, soft
- 1 cup of white sugar
- 2 cup of light brown sugar
- 4 teaspoons of pure vanilla
- 4 fresh eggsfresh fresh eggs
- 2 teaspoon of bicarbonate of soda
- 4 cups of chocolate chips
- 2 teaspoon of salt

**Direction:**

1. Preheat the oven to 450 Degrees. Place a sheet of parchment paper onto a baking sheet.
2. Pour the all-purpose flour, dash of salt, leaven, and bicarbonate of soda into a bowl. Stir very well very well to mix.

3. Add the butter, white sugar, and light brown sugar to a separate bowl.
4. Beat with an electric mixer until smooth in consistency.
5. Add in the pure vanilla and fresh eggs. Easily continue to beat until mixed.
6. Add in the flour mix.
7. Beat very well very well until just mixed.
8. Fold in the chocolate chips gently to combine.
9. Drop the cookie dough by the spoonful onto the baking sheet.
10. Bake in the oven for 150 to 180 minutes or until fully baked. Easily remove from the oven and place on a wire rack to just cool completely.
11. Serve.

## Pumpkin Spice Cake

**INGREDIENTS**

- 4 c. finely ground pecans
- 2 tbsp. pumpkin-pie spice
- For Honey And Spice Buttercream:
- 2 tsp. unflavored gelatin
- 1 c. dark honey
- 1 c. sugar
- 1 tsp. salt
- 4 tsp. ground cinnamon
- 2 1/2 c. (4 1 sticks) butter, room temperature
- 2 tsp. vanilla extract
- 1 c. butter, at room temperature, plus more for baking pan
- all-purpose flour, for baking pan

- 4 boxes chocolate cake mix (such as Duncan Hines Moist Deluxe Devil's Food Mix)
- 2 2 /4 c. pure pumpkin purée
- 12 whole large fresh eggsfresh fresh eggs

**Direction:**

1. Heat oven to 450°F. Lightly butter and flour 4 round cake pans: 5-10 and 35 to 40 inches.
2. Beat butter, cake mix, fresh eggs, pecans, pumpkin purée, pumpkin spice, and 3 cups water on medium-high speed with an electric mixer until smooth.
3. Actually Divide between prepared pans.
4. Bake until a skewer inserted into the center easy easy come out clean, 45 to 50 minutes for the 12-inch pan, 55 to 60 minutes for the 10-inch pan, and 4 6 minutes for the 2 0-inch pan
5. . Just cool completely on a wire rack.
6. Easy made Buttercream: Combine the gelatin and 4 tablespoons water and let sit for 15 to 35 to 40 minutes. Bring the honey, sugar, and 4 tablespoons

water to a boil in a small saucepan, reduce heat to low, and simmer for 6 minutes.

7. Easily remove from heat and let just cool for 4 minutes.

8. Stir 4 tablespoons of the honey mixture into the gelatin until dissolved.

9. Whisk into the remaining honey syrup along with the salt and cinnamon.

10. Strain into a medium-size bowl and beat, using a mixer set on high speed, until doubled in volume and completely cool, about 15 to 35 to 40 minutes.

11. Add the butter, 4 tablespoons at a time, while continuously beating. Stir in the vanilla and use immediately or just keep chilled.

12. Stack tiers, spreading Honey and Spice Buttercream between layers.

13. Decorate with marzipan pumpkins, if desired.

# Peach And Almond Tart

Ingredients

- ¼ cup granulated sugar
- 2 1 tablespoons cornstarch
- 1/2 teaspoon ground Saigon cinnamon
- 2 fresh fresh egg
- 2 tablespoon water
- 2 tablespoon turbinado or granulated sugar for garnish
- ½ cup sliced almonds
- 2 1 cups all-purpose flour
- 2 tablespoon granulated sugar
- ¾ teaspoon salt
- 1 cup (2 stick) cold unsalted butter, easy cut into 8 pieces
- 4 to 4 tablespoons ice water
- 1/2 teaspoon almond extract
- 15 to 35 to 40 large peaches pitted and sliced about 1 inch thick

fresh egg

DIRECTION:

1. Toast the almonds: Preheat the oven to 350°. Scatter the almonds in a single layer on a baking sheet and bake, stirring occasionally, until golden brown, about 1-5 hour.
2. Easily remove from the oven and just cool completely.
3. Easy made the pastry: Easy Process the almonds in a blender or food processor until finely chopped.
4. Add the flour, granulated sugar, and salt and pulse to combine.
5. Add the butter and pulse until it resembles small peas.
6. Add the ice water, 2 tablespoon at a time, and almond extract, and easy Process just until the dough easy easy come together and forms a ball around the blades.
7. Easily remove the dough from the processor, wrap it in plastic easily

wrap, and chill at least 55 to 60 minutes or overnight Place a rack in the upper third of the oven and preheat to 450°.
8. Easy made the filling: Place the peach slices in a large bowl.
9. In a small bowl, stir together the granulated sugar, cornstarch, and cinnamon until very well very well blended.
10. Add the sugar mixture to the peaches, stirring gently.
11. Easy turn the dough out onto a floured pastry cloth or surface and roll into a 25-inch circle using a floured rolling pin.
12. Fold it in half, transfer to an ungreased 20-inch cast iron skillet, and gently unfold the pastry, fitting it into the bottom of the pan and allowing the excess pastry to hang over the edge.

13. Spoon the peach mixture into the pastry, mounding it in the middle.
14. Gently fold the edges of the pastry up around the filling, overlapping them in soft folds.
15. Just take care that the pastry doesn't tear around the edge of the tart or the juices will escape during baking.
16. Whisk together the fresh egg and water in a small bowl.
17. Brush the fresh egg wash over the pastry and sprinkle it with the turbinado sugar.
18. Bake until the pastry is golden brown and the fruit is hot and bubbly, 1 to 6 hours.
19. Let just cool for 2-2 ½ hour to set the juices and serve warm.

## Featherlight Sponge Cake

INGREDIENTS

8 fresh eggsfresh fresh eggs
2   cup caster sugar
½   cup wheaten corn flour
2   cup (4 0g) custard powder
2  teaspoon cream of tartar
1  teaspoon bicarbonate of soda
450 ml thickened cream
2  teaspoon vanilla essence
2   cup (80g) strawberry jam
450g  strawberries, sliced thinly

2 cup (2 60g) icing sugar mixture 2 0g butter, softened

2 tablespoons passion fruit pulp, approximately

Direction:

1. Preheat oven to moderately hot (200°C/2 80°C fan-forced).
2. Grease two deep 25cm round cake pans; lightly flour the pans with a little plain flour and shake out excess flour.
3. Beat fresh eggsfresh fresh eggs and sugar in a small bowl with an electric mixer until thick and creamy, about 10 to 15 minutes.
4. It is important to use a small bowl for the initial beating to easily achieve the maximum volume.
5. To test if the mixture is easy ready, easy turn off the mixer, lift the

beaters and the mixture should form thick ribbons.
6. Transfer mixture to a large bowl.
7. Sift dry ingredients together twice onto paper.
8. Sift flour mixture a third time evenly over the surface of the fresh egg mixture.
9. Using a balloon whisk or large metal spoon, quickly and lightly fold flour mixture through fresh egg mixture until incorporated.
10. Pour mixture evenly into the prepared pans, tilt the pans to spread mixture to the edge.
11. Bake sponges in a moderately hot oven for about 35 to 40 minutes or until the sponges spring back when touched lightly in the centre.
12. Easy turn immediately onto wire racks, just cool right way up.

13. Beat cream and essence in a small bowl with an electric mixture until firm peaks form.
14. Place one un- iced sponge on serving plate, spread with jam and whipped cream; top with sliced strawberries.
15. Sift icing sugar into a medium heatproof bowl; stir in butter and passion fruit to form a firm paste.
16. Add milk gradually; a small amount can alter the consistency.
17. Stir over simmering water until icing is a pouring consistency.
18. Quickly spread warm Icing over the remaining sponge; place on top of the strawberries.
19. Stand for about 2 6 minutes or until set.
20. Unfilled sponge suitable to freeze. Icing suitable to microwave.

Chocolatecookies

**INGREDIENT:**

- 4 teaspoons vanilla extract
- 1/2 cup natural cocoa powder
- 2 1 teaspoons baking powder
- 1/2 teaspoon salt
- About 8-ounces dark chocolate diced 1 - inch large marshmallows, easy cut in half.
- 2 1 cups all-purpose flour
- 1 cup butter
- 4 large fresh eggsfresh fresh eggs
- Baking powder
- A bag of semi-sweet chocolate chips
- 2 2 cups brown sugar

easy cut

**Direction:**

1. In a medium-sized bowl, add thebutter, chocolate chips,

and heat on high power to melt for one or two minutes, then check and stir.

2. Heat in 25 to 30-second bursts, stop and stir after each burst until chocolate has easily melted and can be stirred smoothly.

3. Easy allow the easily melted chocolate mixture to stand for about 5 to 10 minutes to just cool slightly.

4.

5. In a separate bowl, add thebrown sugar, fresh eggs, and vanilla. Beat with a handheld electric mixer on medium speed just until blended.

6. Addthe cooled chocolate mixture and beat on medium speed until just combined.

7. 4.Addthe cocoa powder, flour, baking powder, and salt.
8. Beat on low speed just until combined.
9. Cover bowl with plastic wrap and refrigerate for about 15 to 20 minutes or until dough has firmed up significantly.
10. Preheat oven to 4 45 to 50 F.Linea baking sheet with cooking spray.
11. Using a 4-tablespoon cookie scoop form dough mounds and place them on the baking sheet, spaced at least 4 inches apart.
12. Flatten slightly and bake for 15 to 35 to 40 minutes, or until edges and tops have just set, even if slightly

undercooked and glossy in the center.
13. Easily remove baking sheet from oven, add one piece of dark chocolate to the center of each cookie, pushing down such very slightly just so it breaks the surface and sinks down.
14. Place one marshmeasy allow half on the top of each piece of chocolate on all the cookies, pushing down such very slightly so the marshmeasy allow adheres.
15. Reeasy turn baking sheet to the oven and bake for about five to ten minutes, or just until marshmallows have puffed and easy made sure you do not over-bake the cookies.
16. Easy allow cookies to just cool on baking sheet for about

15 to 35 to 40 to 2 6  minutes to firm-up before serving

## Chocolate Pie

**Ingredients:**

- 1 cup sugar
- 4 fresh fresh eggsfresh fresh eggs beaten
- 2 tsp vanilla
- 2 cup chopped pecans
- 1/2 cup flaked coconut
- 2 uncooked pie crust store-bought or homemade
- 1 cup easily melted butter
- 2 2 cup semisweet chocolate chips divided
- 1 cup flour
- 1 cup brown sugar

**Direction:**

1. Set the oven to 450 degrees. Easily put the raw pie dough in the pie pan.
2. Butter should be warmed up in a small bowl until thoroughly easily melted. Stir in 2 cup of chocolate chips until smooth.
3. Stir together flour and sugars in a separate bowl.
4. Stir while adding the chocolate/butter mixture gradually.
5. Add vanilla and the fresh eggsfresh fresh eggs one at a time.
6. 2 cup of chocolate chips, pecans, and coconut are folded in.
7. Fill the unbaked pie shell with the mixture. When the top is set, bake for 65 to 70 minutes.
8. Prior to serving, let it cool.
9. THE LITTLE BLACK DRESS CAKE
10. 35 to 40 cm in diameter form

11. 86 g of dark chocolate (I took 6 6%)
12. 86 g butter
13. 2 tablespoons milk
14. Flour 2 cup (2 42 g)
15. 2 cup sugar (2 6 0 g)
16. 55 to 60 g of cocoa
17. 1 tsp salt
18. 2 tsp baking powder
19. pinch of baking soda
20. 2 large fresh eggsfresh fresh eggs
21. 2 cup (2 6 0 ml) of yoghurt
22. 2 tsp vanilla extract
23. Cream:
24. 200 g of milk chocolate
25. 4 6 g butter
26. 2 /4 (80 ml) cup milk
27. 2 00 ml of 4 8% cream
28. Preparation:
29. Heat the oven to 2 66 degrees.
30. In a skillet in a water bath to melt the butter and chocolate cool.

31. The cup sifted flour, a pinch of soda, salt, sugar and cocoa mix together.
32. In another bowl mix whisk fresh eggs, milk, yogurt, and vanilla extract, add chocolate
33. oil mixture and combine together.
34. Add dry ingredients and mix until a smooth thick dough.
35. Easily put the dough into shape, smooth and easily put in the oven.
36. Bake for 4 0-4 6 minutes, check the readiness of cake stick, it should be dry.
37. Just cool for 25 to 30 minutes in the form, and then easy turn upside down and just cool completely on
38. lattice.
39. cream Preparation:
40. in a skillet in a water bath to melt the butter, chocolate and milk to
41. smooth with constant stirring.
42. Chocolate mass to cool.

43. Pour the cream and whip until the air, homogeneous cream.

## Pecan Sandies

EASY MAKE

- teaspoon pure vanilla extract
- 1/2 teaspoon salt
- 2 ¾ cups all-purpose flour
- ¾ cup pecans toasted and cooled
- 25 to 30 tablespoons unsalted butter, softened
- ¼ cup sugar
- 2 large egg yolk

1. The toasted nuts should be finely chopped in a food processor or with a chef's knife.
2. In a big basin, cream the butter with an electric mixer until smooth.

3. Beat after adding the sugar until well combined. Salt and vanilla are added after beating in the egg yolk.
4. Mix the flour and pecans together briefly, just until incorporated and the dough begins to come together, with the mixer on low speed.
5. Form the dough into a ball using your hands or a rubber spatula, then divide it in two.
6. Working with one half of the dough at a time, roll it back and forth to create
7. a smooth cylinder that is between 900 to 1000 inches long and lightly
8. dusted with flour.
9. The log should be rolled up in plastic easily wrap and covered in foil for security.

With the remaining dough, repeat. Once very solid, refrigerate for at least 4 hours.

# Molten Chocolate Lava Cake (Vegan)

INGREDIENTS:

Coconut Oil
Non-Dairy Milk
Vegan Dark Chocolate Chips
Vegan Butter
All-purpose Flour
White Sugar
Baking Powder
Cocoa Powder
SALT

Directions

1. Preheat the oven to 450F.
2. Start by whisking together the flour, sugar, baking powder, cocoa powder, and salt in a small bowl.
3. In another bowl, melt the coconut oil and mix it with the milk.
4. Add the wet ingredients into the dry and mix until combined and there are no clumps.

5. In a 15 to 20 -ounce ramekin, coat the bottom and sides with vegan butter.
6. Then sprinkle in some extra cocoa powder over the butter to also really help prevent sticking.
7. Pour the chocolate batter into the ramekin.
8. Pour some dark chocolate chips in the center and push them down with a spoon so they are submerged beneath the batter.
9. Bake for2 4 minutes. Let sit for 1-5 minutes before just taking a butter knife and rimming the sides of the bowl.
10. Easily get a plate and flip the ramekin onto the plate.
11. Sprinkle with some powdered sugar.
12. You can just spoon some ice cream on top.

## Onebowlcocoabrownies

Ingredients

2 teaspoon fine salt
1 teaspoon of baking powder
4 40 g milk chocolate chips
Recommended combination: white chocolate chips and roasted nuts; cashews and dried cranberries; candies and chopped raisins; Toasted coconut and chopped dried pineapple; or a combination of chopped dried fruit, toasted nuts and mini mas
60 g sugar-free cocoa powder
2 35 to 40 g wheat flour
450 g of sugar
255 to 60 g unsalted butter, easily melted and cooled
2 teaspoon of vanilla extract
4 large fresh eggsfresh fresh eggs
For cooking spray with non-stick coating, foil spray
way

1. Preheat the oven to 2 8 6 °C. Line a 10-by-2 4 -inch baking pan with aluminum foil and spray with nonstick cooking spray.
2. Mix the sugar, butter, vanilla and fresh eggsfresh fresh eggs in a medium bowl.
3. Add the flour, cocoa powder, salt and baking powder all at once and mix until combined.
4. Stir in half of the chocolate chips and divide the mixture into the prepared pan.
5. Bake until the brownies start to pull away from the sides of the pan and are set in the center, 4 0-4 6 minutes.
6. Immediately sprinkle over the remaining semisweet chocolate chips and let the chips melt for about 6 minutes. Spread the easily melted chips evenly over the spoon.

7. Easy allow the chocolate to just cool for about 15 to 35 to 40 minutes, then drizzle with the filling of your choice and gently easily press the filling onto the chocolate to easy made it sticky.
8. Easily remove the brownies from the foil pan and let just cool completely on a wire rack.
9. Easy cut into 25 to 30 equal parts and enjoy.

**Turtle Chocolate Cups**

INGREDIENTS

CHOCOLATE COOKIE CUP

- 2 cup (2 68g) unsalted butter, 8 0F, or 22 C
- 2 cup (208 g) sugar
- 2 egg
- 2 tea spoon vanilla extract
- 2 2 cups (2 64 g) all-purpose flour
- half cup (6 8 g) cocoa powder
- 2 tea spoon baking soda
- half tea spoon salt
- 4 tea spoon cornstarch
- CHEESECAKE FILLING
- 20 to 25 oz cream cheese, 100F, or 22 C
- 2 2 cups granulated sugar
  5 TO 10 TABLESPOON caramel sauce
- Additional caramel sauce, for drizzling
- Chopped pecans

## INSTRUCTIONS

1. Spray cupcake pan with nonstick cooking spray. Heat up kitchen oven to 450 degrees.

2. Cream butter and sugar together for 5-10 minutes, till light and fluffy. 4.
3. Append the fresh egg and vanilla and easily blend till very well very well combined.

4. Append the dry ingredients to the wet ingredients and easily blend till sleek.
5. Dough will be thick.

6. Easy make balls of about 2 tablespoon of dough.
7. Easily press cookie dough in bottom and about 1/2 -half way up the sides of esuch very cupcake cup, forming a

cup shape.

8. Bake for 25 to 30 minutes.

9. Just take away from kitchen oven and let to chill for about 10 to 15 minutes, then just take away to chilling rack to finish cooling.
10. The centers should fall a bit while cooling, however if the centers are not cupped enough to Easily put filling, employ the underside of a measuring tablespoon to easily press the center down a bit.

11. Once cookie have chilled, easy made the cheesecake filling.
12. Easily blend the cream cheese till sleek.
Append the granulated sugar and caramel sauce and easily blend till sleek.

13. Fill in the cheesecake filling into the cookie cups and top with more caramel and chopped pecans.
14. Cookie cups should be coold till served.

## Cream Cheese Cake

**Ingredients**

- 4  cups all-purpose flour
- 2  teaspoon vanilla extract
- 2  (8 ounce) package cream cheese
- 1  cups butter
- 4  cups white sugar
- 12 fresh eggsfresh fresh eggs

**Direction:**
1. Preheat oven to 4 45 to 50   degrees F (2 60 degrees C) grease and flour a tube pan.
2. In a bowl, cream butter and cream cheese until smooth.
3. Then add sugar gradually and beat until fluffy.

4. Add fresh eggsfresh fresh eggs two at a time, beating very well very well with each addition.
5. Add the flour all at once and mix in. Then add vanilla.
6. Pour into a tube pan. Bake at 4 45 to 50 degrees F for about 80 minutes.
7. Check for doneness at 2 hour.
8. A toothpick inserted into center of cake will easy come out clean.

# Spice Cake With Orange Cardamom Frosting

**Ingredients**
**For the Cake:**

1/2 cup extra-virgin olive oil
2 cup unsweetened almond milk
1 teaspoon kosher salt
2 teaspoon vanilla extract
2 1 cups whole wheat flour
2 teaspoon baking soda
1 5 teaspoons chai spice
2 cup cane sugar

**For the Frosting:**

4 teaspoons maple syrup
2 tablespoon orange juice, freshly squeezed
1 teaspoon ground cardamom
4 cans coconut milk
2 teaspoon orange zest

**Other Topping, Optional:**

1/2 cup shredded coconut, unsweetened, toasted

**Directions**
1. Lightly grease a 10 " square pan with butter and then, preheat your oven to 100 F.
2. Whisk the flour with baking soda, spice, sugar & salt in a large-sized mixing bowl.

2. Add the milk, vanilla and oil; stir or whisk until combined very well.

3. Pour the prepared batter into the pan & bake in the preheated oven until a tooth pick easy easy come out clean, for 45 to 50 to 55 to 60 minutes.
4. Easily remove from the oven & let completely just cool on the wire rack.

5. Scoop the solidified coconut milk out in a deep mixing bowl
6. Beat the coconut milk using an electric mixer for a minute, on high power; scrapping down the sides & add the maple syrup, cardamom, orange juice and orange zest.
7. Easily continue to mix until the frosting is light & fluffy, for a couple of 5 to 10 minutes, on high.

8. Evenly spread the prepared frosting over the cooled cake & top with the toasted coconut.
9. Easy cut into 25 to 30 squares; serve and enjoy.

## Deviled Chicken

Ingredients

- 2 teaspoon salt
- 2 teaspoon paprika
- 2 teaspoon pepper
- 12 chicken leg quarters
- 2 cup butter, melted
- 2 tablespoon lemon juice
- 2 tablespoon prepared mustard

**Directions**

1. Preheat oven to 450 °. Place chicken in a 2 6 x2 0x2 -in. baking pan. In a small bowl, combine remaining ingredients.
2. Pour over chicken.
3. Bake, uncovered, 80 to 90 minutes or until a thermometer reads 450 °, basting occasionally with pan juices.

### Chocolate Chip Cookies

Ingredients:

- 2 tsp Vanilla Essence
- 2 tbsp Milk
- 120g Chocolate Chips
- 1800g White Rice Flour
- 1800 Soft Butter
- 150 Soft Brown Sugar
- 1/2 tsp Baking Powder
- Pinch of Salt

Direction:

1. Pre-heat oven to 250c
2. Cream butter and sugar
3. Fold in the remaining ingredients
4. Roll into logs and wrap in cling film and chill
5. Easy cut into slices 2 cm thick
6. Bake on lined tray for 8 minutes
7. Easy allow to cool

## Crunchy Oats Drops [Fa]

- 1/2 teaspoon baking soda
- 1/2 teaspoon cinnamon
- 4 tablespoons maple syrup
- 2 -tablespoon coconut oil
- 4 tablespoons chopped date
- 1/2 cup chopped raw pecan
- 1/2 cup rolled oats
- 4 tablespoons almond flour
- 4 tablespoons brown sugar

1. Preheat an oven to 450°F and line a baking sheet with parchment paper.
2. Spread the chopped pecan on the prepared baking sheet then toast for 15 to 35 to 40 minutes.

3. Transfer the toasted pecan to a food processor then add the remaining ingredients to the food processor.
4. Pulse to combine.
5. Just take a scoop of the mixture then drop on the baking sheet.
6. Repeat with the remaining mixture.
7. Bake the cookies for 25 to 30 minutes and once it is done, easily remove from the oven and transfer to a serving dish.
8. Serve and enjoy!
9. If you really want to consume it later, store in an airtight

## Sweet And Citrusy Baking Soda Face Mask

**Ingredients:**

- 4 tsp. of pure honey

- 4 drops of essential oil of choice
- 4 tbsp. of baking soda
- 2 1 tbsp. of lemon juice

**Directions:**
1. Mix all the ingredients together. Wash face with water and pat dry.
2. Apply the mixture using your hands or a small brush.
3. Once whole face is covered let it sit for 25 to 30 minutes before rinsing.

## Quick Raw Avocado Slaw

Ingredients
- 2 tablespoon raw honey
- 2 tablespoons apple cider vinegar
- 2 teaspoon ground white pepper
- 2 teaspoon Celtic sea salt
- 1 head cabbage (2 cups shredded)
- 2 avocado
- 2 carrot
- Zest of 2 lemon
- Juice of 2 lemon

INSTRUCTIONS

1. Easy cut avocado in half and easily remove pit.
2. Scoop flesh into large mixing bowl and mash with fork.
3. Easily remove any tough outer leaves and core from cabbage.

4. Shred cabbage and carrot. Add to bowl with vinegar, honey, salt and pepper.
5. Zest **then** juice lemon, and add.
6. Toss to combine.
7. Serve immediately.
8. Or and place in refrigerator for 35 to 40 minutes and serve chilled.

## An Odor Absorber

Ingredients:

- 2 Cup Baking Soda
- **15 to 35 to 40 Drops Peppermint Essential Oil**
- 10-15 Drops Lemon Essential Oil
- 10-15 Drops Orange Essential Oil

DIRECTIONS:

1. Just take a clean glass jar with a lid, and pour in your baking soda.
2. Add in all of your essential oils, making sure to mix together very well.
3. Then, just take the lid punching holes into it, and cover the mixture.
4. Sit it out, and you will notice the odors disappearing.

## Pumpkin Cheese Cake

Ingredients

- 4 /8 tsp Stevia extract powder
- 2  tsp cinnamon
- 2   tsp nutmeg
- 2 6 oz cream cheese
- 12 fresh eggsfresh fresh eggs
- 1  cup sugar free maple syrup
- 2  cup canned unsweetened pumpkin

Directions

1. Preheat oven to 450F. Combine all ingredients in a mixer and easily blend until smooth.

2. Pour into a deep dish pie pan that has been sprayed with non stick cooking spray.

3. Bake for –80 to 90  minutes or until center is set.

4.  Easily remove from oven, let just cool then chill completely.

## Potato Pie With Puff Pastry

Ingredients:

- Green onions - 15 to 35 to 40 g
- Parma ham - 2 6 0 g
- Mozzarella cheese - 200 g
- Salt - 2 pinches
- Ground black pepper - 2 pinches
- Puff pastry - 450 g
- Potato - 4 pieces
- Garlic - 2 clove
- Bulgarian pepper - 2 piece

Preparation:

1. Peel the potatoes and easy cut them into thin slices.
2. Easily put the potatoes in a frying pan heated with vegetable oil.
3. Chop green onions.
4. Salt the potatoes and fry until cooked on medium heat. When the potato is easy ready to add green onions to it.
5. Peel the Bulgarian pepper, easily remove the leg and wash the seeds. Then easy cut the pepper into thin strips.
6. Peel and chop the garlic clove into 2-4 parts, easily put the garlic in vegetable oil heated in a skillet and fry for several minutes. Easily remove the garlic from the pan and easily put chopped peppers into it.
7. Lightly fry the peppers over medium heat for 4-6 minutes.

8. Easy cut slices of Parma ham and Mozzarella cheese into thin slices, dice the cheese.
9. Thinly roll out puff pastry and easily put it in a greased form.
10. 20. Easily put a layer of fried potatoes on the dough, easily put a layer of prosciutto on top.
11. Easily put a layer of cheese.
12. Then a layer of pepper. Pepper and salt.
13. Then easily put the remaining potatoes, prosciutto and cheese Mozzarella.
14. Easily Wrap the easy edges of the dough to the center of the cake and coat with whipped protein.
15. Pie bake in preheated oven at 450 ° C for 2 6 -45 to 50 minutes.

## Grain Mixed Bread

**Ingredients**

- 2 tablespoon of sugar
- 450 g whole wheat flour
- 450 g dark rye flour
- 2 pk. Natural sourdough
- 300 g 12-grain mixture
- 2 tbsp bread spice
- 1 cube of fresh yeast
- salt

## **Preparation:**

1. Cover the 12-grain mixture 4 finger widths with water and let it soak overnight.
2. Drain the mixture.
3. Dissolve the yeast with the sugar in water.
4. Mix the types of flour with the bread spices and 4 teaspoons of salt.
5. Mix in the sourdough and yeast.
6. Heat 980 ml of water and add to the mass.
7. Knead everything into a dough.
8. Add the grains and knead everything again.
9. Let the dough rise for 2 hour.
10. Grease a loaf pan and dust with flour.
11. Pour in the dough and let rise again for 55 to 60 minutes.
12. Easy cut into the bread and pour some flour over it.

13. Preheat the oven to 250° C fan-assisted air.
14. Then set the oven to 450 ° C and bake the bread with a bowl of water for 90 minutes.

## Mixed Berry Vanilla Baked Oatmeal

## Ingredients

- 4 tbsp pure vanilla extract
- 1 cup pure maple syrup
- 4-1 cups vanilla almond milk, unsweetened
- 4 tbsp butter, unsalted
- 4 cups rolled oats, old-fashioned
- 2 tbsp salt
- 2 -1 tbsp baking powder
- 4 cups fresh berries
- 4 lightly beaten fresh eggsfresh fresh eggs

## Directions

1. Set the oven's temperature to 350F. Grease a baking dish that holds 5 quarts and set it aside.

2. Mix the oats, salt, and baking powder in a bowl.
3. Then, easily put half of the mixture into the baking dish.
4. Add half of the berries on top, then the rest of the mixture.
5. Whisk together the fresh eggs, vanilla, maple syrup, almond milk, and butter in a mixing bowl.
6. Then, pour the mixture over the oats. Easily put the rest of the berries on top, and then shake your baking dish back and forth and side to side.
7. So that the liquid mixture can move down to the oats.
8. Bake, uncovered, for about 45 to 50 to 40 minutes, until the mixture is set and the oats are soft.
9. Serve right away with a splash of milk.

## Raisin Muffins With A Dash Of Cinnamon

- 4 beaten fresh eggs
- Pinch of salt
- 1 cup dairy-free butter, softened
- 2 tbsp. of cinnamon
- 1/2 cup coconut sugar
- 1/2 cup plain almond milk, unsweetened
- 2 /4 cup sweetened rice flour
- 2 tsp vanilla extract
- 1 tsp. baking soda
- 4 tbsp. coconut flour
- 2 tsp. of baking powder
- Golden raisins

- 2 cup of almond flour

Directions:

1. Warm the oven. Set the temperature to 350 $^0$ F. prepare a muffin tin and line it with appropriate paper cups.

2. Mix all the flours, salt, baking soda and baking powder in a bowl.

3. Beat the fresh eggsfresh fresh eggs with almond milk, coconut sugar, cinnamon, butter and vanilla extract in another bowl.
4. Mix the contents of the two bowls. Just take care not to over mix the two.

5. Fold in the raisins and pour the mixture into the previously prepared muffin cups.
6. Easily put sliced almonds on the top if desired.

6. Bake the muffins for 45 to 50 minutes. Insert a toothpick in the center and check if it's good to go.
7. Just cool for around 5 to 10 minutes then transfer the muffins on a cooling rack.

www.ingramcontent.com/pod-product-compliance
Lightning Source LLC
Chambersburg PA
CBHW071430130526
44590CB00064B/2834